Medical Memories

My Personal Medical Tracker

EZLifeTrackers.com

Created: By Steve Mitchell

Copyright © 2019, by SMF Services, Inc.

ISBN: 9781661367794

We all go to doctors. Each of us has different health issues or circumstances. **Sometimes the doctor may ask us to track certain factors while other times we may decide to do the tracking for our own personal reasons.**

We have made EZ Life Trackers for some of the many popular places throughout the world and for many of the activities in life, like our everyday health.

DO YOU HAVE A GREAT MEMORY? Most of us need reminders…

This EZ Life Tracker is 8.5" x 11" with a total of 100 pages, 98 for data entry.

Medical Memories enables you to record important health information like Your Medical History, Your Mother's Medical History, Your Father's Medical History, Your Medications and Dosage, Your Doctors and Specialists, The Hospitals that you have used, Your Operations, Your Testing History, Medication Tracking, Weight Tracking, Blood Pressure Tracking, Pain Tracking and the recording of other General Health issues and concerns.

The General Health areas can be used if there are not enough specific areas for your needs. All sections should be updated as appropriate to help you to maintain an accurate record of your health.

Extend your memory. Also, provide a great resource for your doctors and family when needed by maintaining a regularly updated Medical Memories, My Personal Medical Tracker.

Best of luck and I hope that this EZ Life Tracker proves to be an invaluable resource and record for you during a hopefully healthy life.

Medical Memories, My Personal Medical Tracker is provided courtesy of:

_____
_____
_____
_____
_____

EZ Life Trackers-For A Better Documented Life!

www.ezlifetrackers.com

Medical History

Patient Name: _____

Age: ____ Sex: _____ Marital Status: _____

Known Medical Conditions & History:
_____
_____
_____
_____
_____
_____
_____
_____
_____
_____
_____
_____
_____
_____
_____
_____
_____
_____
_____
_____
_____
_____
_____

Mother's Known Medical Conditions:
_____
_____
_____
_____
_____
_____
_____
_____

Father's Known Medical Conditions:
_____
_____
_____
_____
_____

Grandmother's Medical Conditions:
_____
_____
_____
_____
_____

Grandfather's Medical Conditions:
_____
_____
_____
_____
_____

List Medications

(Cross Off The Medication When You Stop Taking It)

Medication	Dose	Medication	Dose

List Medications

(Cross Off The Medication When You Stop Taking It)

Medication	Dose	Medication	Dose

Doctors

Primary: (Include Name, Address & Telephone Number (Update Over Time):

_____
_____
_____
_____
_____

Specialists: (Include Name, Address & Telephone Number (Update Over Time):

_____
_____
_____
_____
_____
_____
_____
_____
_____
_____

Medical Insurance: (Include Company and Policy Number)

_____
_____
_____
_____
_____
_____
_____
_____
_____
_____

Hospitals Used In Past: (Include Dates and Reason):

_____
_____
_____
_____
_____
_____
_____
_____
_____

Major Operations:

(Include What Was Done, Dates & Times)

_____
_____
_____
_____
_____
_____
_____
_____
_____
_____
_____
_____
_____
_____
_____
_____

Major Operations:

(Include What Was Done, Dates & Times)

_____
_____
_____
_____
_____
_____
_____
_____
_____
_____
_____
_____
_____
_____
_____
_____
_____
_____
_____
_____
_____
_____
_____
_____
_____
_____
_____
_____
_____
_____
_____
_____

Lab Tests, EKGs, ECOs, X-rays & Other Testing:

(Include Dates & Where)

EZ Medication Tracker

Medication	Dose	Date	Time	Doctor

EZ Medication Tracker

Medication	Dose	Date	Time	Doctor

EZ Medication Tracker

Medication	Dose	Date	Time	Doctor

EZ Medication Tracker

Medication	Dose	Date	Time	Doctor

EZ Medication Tracker

Medication	Dose	Date	Time	Doctor

EZ Medication Tracker

Medication	Dose	Date	Time	Doctor

EZ Medication Tracker

Medication	Dose	Date	Time	Doctor

EZ Medication Tracker

Medication	Dose	Date	Time	Doctor

EZ Medication Tracker

Medication	Dose	Date	Time	Doctor

EZ Medication Tracker

Medication	Dose	Date	Time	Doctor

EZ Weight Tracker

	Date	Weight	Time	Comments / Notes
1				
2				
3				
4				
5				
6				
7				
8				
9				
10				
11				
12				
13				
14				
15				
16				
17				
18				
19				
20				
21				
22				
23				
24				
25				
26				
27				
28				
29				
30				
31				

EZ Weight Tracker

	Date	Weight	Time	Comments / Notes
1				
2				
3				
4				
5				
6				
7				
8				
9				
10				
11				
12				
13				
14				
15				
16				
17				
18				
19				
20				
21				
22				
23				
24				
25				
26				
27				
28				
29				
30				
31				

EZ Weight Tracker

	Date	Weight	Time	Comments / Notes
1				
2				
3				
4				
5				
6				
7				
8				
9				
10				
11				
12				
13				
14				
15				
16				
17				
18				
19				
20				
21				
22				
23				
24				
25				
26				
27				
28				
29				
30				
31				

EZ Weight Tracker

	Date	Weight	Time	Comments / Notes
1				
2				
3				
4				
5				
6				
7				
8				
9				
10				
11				
12				
13				
14				
15				
16				
17				
18				
19				
20				
21				
22				
23				
24				
25				
26				
27				
28				
29				
30				
31				

EZ Weight Tracker

	Date	Weight	Time	Comments / Notes
1				
2				
3				
4				
5				
6				
7				
8				
9				
10				
11				
12				
13				
14				
15				
16				
17				
18				
19				
20				
21				
22				
23				
24				
25				
26				
27				
28				
29				
30				
31				

EZ Weight Tracker

	Date	Weight	Time	Comments / Notes
1				
2				
3				
4				
5				
6				
7				
8				
9				
10				
11				
12				
13				
14				
15				
16				
17				
18				
19				
20				
21				
22				
23				
24				
25				
26				
27				
28				
29				
30				
31				

EZ Blood Pressure Tracker

Date	Time	Systolic	Diastolic	Date	Time	Systolic	Diastolic

EZ Blood Pressure Tracker

Date	Time	Systolic	Diastolic	Date	Time	Systolic	Diastolic

EZ Blood Pressure Tracker

Date	Time	Systolic	Diastolic	Date	Time	Systolic	Diastolic

EZ Blood Pressure Tracker

Date	Time	Systolic	Diastolic	Date	Time	Systolic	Diastolic

EZ Blood Pressure Tracker

Date	Time	Systolic	Diastolic	Date	Time	Systolic	Diastolic

EZ Blood Pressure Tracker

Date	Time	Systolic	Diastolic	Date	Time	Systolic	Diastolic

EZ Blood Pressure Tracker

Date	Time	Systolic	Diastolic	Date	Time	Systolic	Diastolic

EZ Blood Pressure Tracker

Date	Time	Systolic	Diastolic	Date	Time	Systolic	Diastolic

Pain Tracking

Pain Start Date: _____ Pain Start Time: _____ Pain End Time: _____ Duration: ___

Pain Description:
_____
_____
_____
_____
_____

Pain Severity: 1 2 3 4 5 6 7 8 9 10

Medication(s) Taken:
_____
_____
_____
_____

Treatment:
_____
_____
_____
_____
_____
_____
_____
_____

Effects of Treatment:
_____
_____
_____
_____
_____
_____

Pain Tracking

Pain Start Date: _____ Pain Start Time: _____ Pain End Time: _____ Duration: ____

Pain Description:

_____
_____
_____
_____
_____

Pain Severity: 1 2 3 4 5 6 7 8 9 10

Medication(s) Taken:

_____
_____
_____
_____

Treatment:

_____
_____
_____
_____
_____
_____
_____
_____

Effects of Treatment:

_____
_____
_____
_____
_____
_____

Pain Tracking

Pain Start Date: _____ Pain Start Time: _____ Pain End Time: _____ Duration: ____

Pain Description:
_____
_____
_____
_____
_____

Pain Severity: 1 2 3 4 5 6 7 8 9 10

Medication(s) Taken:
_____
_____
_____
_____

Treatment:
_____
_____
_____
_____
_____
_____
_____
_____
_____

Effects of Treatment:
_____
_____
_____
_____
_____
_____

Pain Tracking

Pain Start Date: _____ Pain Start Time: _____ Pain End Time: _____ Duration: ___

Pain Description:
_____
_____
_____
_____
_____

Pain Severity: 1 2 3 4 5 6 7 8 9 10

Medication(s) Taken:
_____
_____
_____
_____

Treatment:
_____
_____
_____
_____
_____
_____
_____
_____

Effects of Treatment:
_____
_____
_____
_____
_____
_____

Pain Tracking

Pain Start Date: _____ Pain Start Time: _____ Pain End Time: _____ Duration: ___

Pain Description:
_____
_____
_____
_____
_____

Pain Severity: 1 2 3 4 5 6 7 8 9 10

Medication(s) Taken:
_____
_____
_____
_____

Treatment:
_____
_____
_____
_____
_____
_____
_____

Effects of Treatment:
_____
_____
_____
_____
_____

Pain Tracking

Pain Start Date: _____ Pain Start Time: _____ Pain End Time: _____ Duration: ____

Pain Description:
_____
_____
_____
_____
_____

Pain Severity: 1 2 3 4 5 6 7 8 9 10

Medication(s) Taken:
_____
_____
_____
_____

Treatment:
_____
_____
_____
_____
_____
_____
_____
_____

Effects of Treatment:
_____
_____
_____
_____
_____

Pain Tracking

Pain Start Date: _____   Pain Start Time: _____   Pain End Time: _____   Duration: ____

Pain Description:

_____
_____
_____
_____
_____

Pain Severity: 1   2   3   4   5   6   7   8   9   10

Medication(s) Taken:

_____
_____
_____
_____

Treatment:

_____
_____
_____
_____
_____
_____
_____
_____

Effects of Treatment:

_____
_____
_____
_____
_____
_____

Pain Tracking

Pain Start Date: _____ Pain Start Time: _____ Pain End Time: _____ Duration: ___

Pain Description:
_____
_____
_____
_____
_____

Pain Severity: 1 2 3 4 5 6 7 8 9 10

Medication(s) Taken:
_____
_____
_____
_____

Treatment:
_____
_____
_____
_____
_____
_____
_____
_____

Effects of Treatment:
_____
_____
_____
_____
_____

Pain Tracking

Pain Start Date: _____ Pain Start Time: _____ Pain End Time: _____ Duration: ___

Pain Description:
_____
_____
_____
_____
_____

Pain Severity: 1 2 3 4 5 6 7 8 9 10

Medication(s) Taken:
_____
_____
_____
_____

Treatment:
_____
_____
_____
_____
_____
_____
_____
_____

Effects of Treatment:
_____
_____
_____
_____
_____
_____

Pain Tracking

Pain Start Date: _____ Pain Start Time: _____ Pain End Time: _____ Duration: ____

Pain Description:
_____
_____
_____
_____
_____

Pain Severity: 1 2 3 4 5 6 7 8 9 10

Medication(s) Taken:
_____
_____
_____
_____

Treatment:
_____
_____
_____
_____
_____
_____
_____
_____

Effects of Treatment:
_____
_____
_____
_____
_____
_____

Pain Tracking

Pain Start Date: _____ Pain Start Time: _____ Pain End Time: _____ Duration: ____

Pain Description:
_____
_____
_____
_____
_____

Pain Severity: 1 2 3 4 5 6 7 8 9 10

Medication(s) Taken:
_____
_____
_____
_____

Treatment:
_____
_____
_____
_____
_____
_____
_____
_____

Effects of Treatment:
_____
_____
_____
_____
_____
_____

Pain Tracking

Pain Start Date: _____ Pain Start Time: _____ Pain End Time: _____ Duration: ___

Pain Description:
_____
_____
_____
_____
_____

Pain Severity: 1 2 3 4 5 6 7 8 9 10

Medication(s) Taken:
_____
_____
_____
_____

Treatment:
_____
_____
_____
_____
_____
_____
_____
_____

Effects of Treatment:
_____
_____
_____
_____
_____

Pain Tracking

Pain Start Date: _____ Pain Start Time: _____ Pain End Time: _____ Duration: ____

Pain Description:
_____
_____
_____
_____
_____

Pain Severity: 1 2 3 4 5 6 7 8 9 10

Medication(s) Taken:
_____
_____
_____
_____

Treatment:
_____
_____
_____
_____
_____
_____
_____
_____

Effects of Treatment:
_____
_____
_____
_____
_____
_____
_____

Pain Tracking

Pain Start Date: _____ Pain Start Time: _____ Pain End Time: _____ Duration: ____

Pain Description:
_____
_____
_____
_____
_____

Pain Severity: 1 2 3 4 5 6 7 8 9 10

Medication(s) Taken:
_____
_____
_____
_____

Treatment:
_____
_____
_____
_____
_____
_____
_____
_____

Effects of Treatment:
_____
_____
_____
_____
_____
_____
_____
_____

General Health Issues

Health Issues Worth Recording: (Include More Pain and Other Tracking If Needed)

General Health Issues

Health Issues Worth Recording: (Include More Pain and Other Tracking If Needed)

General Health Issues

Health Issues Worth Recording: (Include More Pain and Other Tracking If Needed)

General Health Issues

Health Issues Worth Recording: (Include More Pain and Other Tracking If Needed)

General Health Issues

Health Issues Worth Recording: (Include More Pain and Other Tracking If Needed)
_____
_____
_____
_____
_____
_____
_____
_____
_____
_____
_____
_____
_____
_____
_____
_____
_____
_____
_____
_____
_____
_____
_____
_____
_____
_____
_____
_____
_____
_____
_____
_____
_____
_____
_____
_____
_____
_____
_____
_____

General Health Issues

Health Issues Worth Recording: (Include More Pain and Other Tracking If Needed)

General Health Issues

Health Issues Worth Recording: (Include More Pain and Other Tracking If Needed)
_____
_____
_____
_____
_____
_____
_____
_____
_____
_____
_____
_____
_____
_____
_____
_____
_____
_____
_____
_____
_____
_____
_____
_____
_____
_____
_____
_____
_____
_____
_____
_____

General Health Issues

Health Issues Worth Recording: (Include More Pain and Other Tracking If Needed)

_____
_____
_____
_____
_____
_____
_____
_____
_____
_____
_____
_____
_____
_____
_____
_____
_____
_____
_____
_____
_____
_____
_____
_____
_____
_____
_____
_____
_____
_____

General Health Issues

Health Issues Worth Recording: (Include More Pain and Other Tracking If Needed)
_____
_____
_____
_____
_____
_____
_____
_____
_____
_____
_____
_____
_____
_____
_____
_____
_____
_____
_____
_____
_____
_____
_____
_____
_____
_____
_____
_____
_____
_____
_____
_____

General Health Issues

Health Issues Worth Recording: (Include More Pain and Other Tracking If Needed)
_____
_____
_____
_____
_____
_____
_____
_____
_____
_____
_____
_____
_____
_____
_____
_____
_____
_____
_____
_____
_____
_____
_____
_____
_____
_____
_____
_____
_____
_____
_____
_____
_____
_____
_____
_____

General Health Issues

Health Issues Worth Recording: (Include More Pain and Other Tracking If Needed)

General Health Issues

Health Issues Worth Recording: (Include More Pain and Other Tracking If Needed)
_____
_____
_____
_____
_____
_____
_____
_____
_____
_____
_____
_____
_____
_____
_____
_____
_____
_____
_____
_____
_____
_____
_____
_____
_____
_____
_____
_____
_____
_____

General Health Issues

Health Issues Worth Recording: (Include More Pain and Other Tracking If Needed)

General Health Issues

Health Issues Worth Recording: (Include More Pain and Other Tracking If Needed)

General Health Issues

Health Issues Worth Recording: (Include More Pain and Other Tracking If Needed)
___

General Health Issues

Health Issues Worth Recording: (Include More Pain and Other Tracking If Needed)

General Health Issues

Health Issues Worth Recording: (Include More Pain and Other Tracking If Needed)
_____
_____
_____
_____
_____
_____
_____
_____
_____
_____
_____
_____
_____
_____
_____
_____
_____
_____
_____
_____
_____
_____
_____
_____
_____
_____
_____
_____
_____
_____
_____
_____

General Health Issues

Health Issues Worth Recording: (Include More Pain and Other Tracking If Needed)
___

General Health Issues

Health Issues Worth Recording: (Include More Pain and Other Tracking If Needed)
_____
_____
_____
_____
_____
_____
_____
_____
_____
_____
_____
_____
_____
_____
_____
_____
_____
_____
_____
_____
_____
_____
_____
_____
_____
_____
_____
_____
_____
_____
_____
_____
_____
_____
_____
_____
_____

General Health Issues

Health Issues Worth Recording: (Include More Pain and Other Tracking If Needed)

General Health Issues

Health Issues Worth Recording: (Include More Pain and Other Tracking If Needed)

_____
_____
_____
_____
_____
_____
_____
_____
_____
_____
_____
_____
_____
_____
_____
_____
_____
_____
_____
_____
_____
_____
_____
_____
_____
_____
_____
_____
_____
_____
_____
_____
_____
_____
_____

General Health Issues

Health Issues Worth Recording: (Include More Pain and Other Tracking If Needed)

General Health Issues

Health Issues Worth Recording: (Include More Pain and Other Tracking If Needed)
_____
_____
_____
_____
_____
_____
_____
_____
_____
_____
_____
_____
_____
_____
_____
_____
_____
_____
_____
_____
_____
_____
_____
_____
_____
_____
_____
_____
_____
_____
_____
_____

General Health Issues

Health Issues Worth Recording: (Include More Pain and Other Tracking If Needed)

General Health Issues

Health Issues Worth Recording: (Include More Pain and Other Tracking If Needed)

General Health Issues

Health Issues Worth Recording: (Include More Pain and Other Tracking If Needed)
_____
_____
_____
_____
_____
_____
_____
_____
_____
_____
_____
_____
_____
_____
_____
_____
_____
_____
_____
_____
_____
_____
_____
_____
_____
_____
_____
_____
_____
_____
_____

General Health Issues

Health Issues Worth Recording: (Include More Pain and Other Tracking If Needed)

General Health Issues

Health Issues Worth Recording: (Include More Pain and Other Tracking If Needed)

General Health Issues

Health Issues Worth Recording: (Include More Pain and Other Tracking If Needed)

_____
_____
_____
_____
_____
_____
_____
_____
_____
_____
_____
_____
_____
_____
_____
_____
_____
_____
_____
_____
_____
_____
_____
_____
_____
_____
_____
_____
_____
_____
_____
_____
_____
_____
_____
_____
_____
_____
_____

General Health Issues

Health Issues Worth Recording: (Include More Pain and Other Tracking If Needed)

General Health Issues

Health Issues Worth Recording: (Include More Pain and Other Tracking If Needed)
_____
_____
_____
_____
_____
_____
_____
_____
_____
_____
_____
_____
_____
_____
_____
_____
_____
_____
_____
_____
_____
_____
_____
_____
_____
_____
_____
_____
_____
_____
_____
_____
_____
_____

General Health Issues

Health Issues Worth Recording: (Include More Pain and Other Tracking If Needed)
___
___
___
___
___
___
___
___
___
___
___
___
___
___
___
___
___
___
___
___
___
___
___
___
___
___
___
___
___
___
___
___
___

General Health Issues

Health Issues Worth Recording: (Include More Pain and Other Tracking If Needed)

General Health Issues

Health Issues Worth Recording: (Include More Pain and Other Tracking If Needed)

_____
_____
_____
_____
_____
_____
_____
_____
_____
_____
_____
_____
_____
_____
_____
_____
_____
_____
_____
_____
_____
_____
_____
_____
_____
_____
_____
_____
_____
_____
_____
_____

General Health Issues

Health Issues Worth Recording: (Include More Pain and Other Tracking If Needed)

General Health Issues

Health Issues Worth Recording: (Include More Pain and Other Tracking If Needed)

_____
_____
_____
_____
_____
_____
_____
_____
_____
_____
_____
_____
_____
_____
_____
_____
_____
_____
_____
_____
_____
_____
_____
_____
_____
_____
_____
_____
_____
_____

General Health Issues

Health Issues Worth Recording: (Include More Pain and Other Tracking If Needed)

General Health Issues

Health Issues Worth Recording: (Include More Pain and Other Tracking If Needed)
___

General Health Issues

Health Issues Worth Recording: (Include More Pain and Other Tracking If Needed)
___
___
___
___
___
___
___
___
___
___
___
___
___
___
___
___
___
___
___
___
___
___
___
___
___
___
___
___
___
___
___
___
___
___
___

General Health Issues

Health Issues Worth Recording: (Include More Pain and Other Tracking If Needed)

General Health Issues

Health Issues Worth Recording: (Include More Pain and Other Tracking If Needed)

General Health Issues

Health Issues Worth Recording: (Include More Pain and Other Tracking If Needed)
_____
_____
_____
_____
_____
_____
_____
_____
_____
_____
_____
_____
_____
_____
_____
_____
_____
_____
_____
_____
_____
_____
_____
_____
_____
_____
_____
_____
_____
_____

General Health Issues

Health Issues Worth Recording: (Include More Pain and Other Tracking If Needed)
_____
_____
_____
_____
_____
_____
_____
_____
_____
_____
_____
_____
_____
_____
_____
_____
_____
_____
_____
_____
_____
_____
_____
_____
_____
_____
_____
_____
_____
_____
_____
_____
_____
_____

General Health Issues

Health Issues Worth Recording: (Include More Pain and Other Tracking If Needed)

General Health Issues

Health Issues Worth Recording: (Include More Pain and Other Tracking If Needed)

General Health Issues

Health Issues Worth Recording: (Include More Pain and Other Tracking If Needed)

General Health Issues

Health Issues Worth Recording: (Include More Pain and Other Tracking If Needed)

General Health Issues

Health Issues Worth Recording: (Include More Pain and Other Tracking If Needed)
_____
_____
_____
_____
_____
_____
_____
_____
_____
_____
_____
_____
_____
_____
_____
_____
_____
_____
_____
_____
_____
_____
_____
_____
_____
_____
_____
_____
_____
_____
_____
_____

General Health Issues

Health Issues Worth Recording: (Include More Pain and Other Tracking If Needed)

_____
_____
_____
_____
_____
_____
_____
_____
_____
_____
_____
_____
_____
_____
_____
_____
_____
_____
_____
_____
_____
_____
_____
_____
_____
_____
_____
_____
_____
_____

General Health Issues

Health Issues Worth Recording: (Include More Pain and Other Tracking If Needed)
___
___
___
___
___
___
___
___
___
___
___
___
___
___
___
___
___
___
___
___
___
___
___
___
___
___
___
___
___
___
___
___
___

General Health Issues

Health Issues Worth Recording: (Include More Pain and Other Tracking If Needed)

www.ingramcontent.com/pod-product-compliance
Lightning Source LLC
Chambersburg PA
CBHW081447220526
45466CB00008B/2534